# The Candida Diet Solution

Sandra Boehner

SANDRA BOEHNER

ISBN-10: 147823203X
ISBN-13: 978-1478232032

# DEDICATION

This book is for YOU!

For your trust in me
and your belief in Natural Healing

SANDRA BOEHNER

SANDRA BOEHNER

# CONTENTS

SANDRA BOEHNER

# ACKNOWLEDGMENTS

A big thanks to my long suffering partner Johnny who was at my side during my 4 years long soul destroying recovery from candida, who had to patiently read through numerous early versions of this e-book, who designed the awesome cover for it as well, who solved all my web and formatting related heartaches and who has been my love and best friend for over eight years now.

Thanks must also go to my wonderful parents, Dieter and Inge Böhner, who never lost faith in me despite all set-backs and difficulties. And who instilled the belief in me that good things will come to those who are patient and work hard for it.

Lots of love and thanks go to my partner's parents, Jackie and Terry Pope, who accompanied me through thick and thin, right from the start.

Another big thanks goes to my mentor Cathy Presland for shepherding this book through its various hoops and barrels and helping me to clarify the direction of my business in general.

Next at bat is my dear friend Rebecca Jenkins. Her healing Shiatsu and Japanese style Zen Yoga were crucial to healing my body's imbalances and brought peace to my stressed mind and soul.

I also want to thank Julie Edmonson for doing a stellar job editing out the Cornish-German slang in the manuscript to this e-book.

Thanks to naturopath and herbalists Sara Southgate and Alisha Forbes, who double-checked that the information in this e-book makes medicinal sense.

A massive thanks also goes to all my blog readers and fellow foodie bloggers who are keeping me sane with their health wisdom, their charming comments and their inspiring recipe creations.

Especially Heather from Gluten free Cat, who was one of the first people to kindly offer to review my book on her popular blog.

Many people have in some way helped me on this journey - too many to mention here by name. So don't be sad if I haven't mentioned you this time - there's always my next book, right. So, thanks for reading this far. You're awesome!

## DISCLAIMER

The medical information provided in this e-book cannot substitute the advice of a medical professional e.g. a qualified doctor/ physician. The author herself is no doctor and can therefore not accept any responsibility for the results or consequences if you adopt any of the information in this e-book or on the author's website http://candidadietplan.com.

In an attempt to make the information in the book as medicinally correct as possible the author ran the plan outlined in the book past two naturopaths who said the following:

*"The natural method described in this book seems like a very good way of curing Candida."*

- Sara Southgate BSc., ND, Dip Herb, MURHP

*"For people suffering with candida, this is an invaluable resource that is readily accessible, well researched and covers the most important areas that need to be addressed for healing candida. I commend Sandra for putting so much time and effort into this as it will no doubt be the saviour for so many people needing to address this very common problem"*

- Alisha Lynch, Naturopath

With this legally required note out of the way – let's look at how you can cure candida.

THE CANDIDA DIET SOLUTION

# INTRODUCTION

Have you ever felt completely confused by all the information surrounding the Candida diet? I know I have!

Have you ever been totally frustrated by the amount of conflicting information available out there? Me too!

I've written this book because I know from my own experience how confusing and disheartening it can be in the beginning.

You see, I wished I'd had someone to hold me by the hand and tell me what each phase of the diet is like -- someone to tell me what I should and shouldn't eat and to offer me motivation and encouragement when times got tough.

Instead, I spent 1.5 years figuring things out myself, piecing bits of information together that worked while discarding the rest. I started a blog and a Facebook group ("Detox Buddies"), which now have more than 1,000 followers combined. I met some amazing people who have shared their own Candida stories and health tips with me, and this is what I will share with you!

This e-book is a concise document that brings together my own personal knowledge plus that of hundreds of other sufferers like you. I will walk you through each stage of the Candida diet plan, showing you exactly what you need to do to get yourself back to a full and healthy life!

I intend to put the recipes that I link to in this book into a separate handy little e-book. For now, you can access them from the book or directly through my website.

My heart goes out to you -- living with Candida (even if you just live with somebody who has it) is always a royal pain in the backside. But I am confident that, because you picked up this book and are ready to tackle your health problems, you're only one step away from feeling much better than you have in years.

Well done, you! Keep the momentum going -- drop me a line and tell me how you're doing. I'd love to hear from you!

# CHAPTER ONE

## ABOUT CANDIDA

**What is Candida?**

Candida is an infection caused by a yeast organism (also known as Candida albicans) that is always present in the body. Believe it or not, everyone has yeast growing in their bodies -- even you! Some people never display Candida symptoms because they have immune systems able to cap the yeast growth at a healthy level.

However, others aren't so lucky – some react negatively to Candida and become ill. While it may sound gross, it's a natural, healthy part of the digestive process. Basically, these "friendly bacteria" are the same you see in many yoghurt advertisements. They are essential for your health and take up space in your gut that the yeast might otherwise take over, which is what makes some people sick.

What most people don't realize is that Candida can occur anywhere in the body. And everyone can get it -- both men and women. Even babies can have it in the form of nappy rash. As you're reading this book, I'm presuming you might have it too. Don't worry; we'll get to that in a minute.

More often than not, Candida inflammations are mistaken for other health problems. Colds, runny noses, sneezing and feeling drained are very common signs of Candida!

Unfortunately, these types of symptoms are so common that everyone seems to suffer from them at some point, which is exactly why Candida is often misdiagnosed or unnoticed altogether.

Let me guess. You haven't been feeling well for some time, too, right?

One thing is certain. Candida inflammations are made worse by foods that contain sugar.

**CANDIDA DIET RULE No. 1:**

*Don't eat sweets or any other food that contains sugar.*

**What makes a normal diet not suitable for Candida sufferers?**

When your immune system is already working overtime, eating certain foods can sometimes tip it over the edge. You might find yourself sniffing, sneezing and rubbing your eyes. Having a bloated, aching tummy and/or feeling low are indications of a typical case of food allergy or even leaky gut syndrome.

Why does your body do this? Often times, our bodies send out warning signals well before we get seriously ill. We just have to listen. So if you've been feeling low for some time and regularly find yourself suffering from infections or allergies, it's time to stop asking yourself, "Why do I always get..." Instead, say to yourself, *""Hey, something is not right here. I'm going to give my body time to sort it out. How can I best do this?"*

The answer is by giving your digestive system a rest so that the energy normally spent on digesting food can now be used to heal you. And no, your body doesn't automatically digest food.

Believe me, it does spend a lot of energy on it -- just in the background without you noticing it! This is where the Candida diet comes in.

## CANDIDA DIET RULE No. 2

*The basic idea behind the Candida diet is simple -- to eliminate foods that don't agree with you!*

### Three types of food that are eliminated during the Candida diet:

### 1. Allergens

Foods that you could be allergic to or intolerant of (e.g., milk, nuts, oats, wheat).

### 2. Sugar

Foods that promote yeast growth (i.e., anything containing sugar, yeast or fermented ingredients).

### 3. Heavy Food

Foods that are really hard to digest or sit in your digestive system for a long time (e.g., dark meat and greasy, fried and very spicy food).

I have put together a list of foods you can and can't eat for each stage of the Candida diet. There are four stages (but we'll get to that in a minute).

Did you know that more than 75 percent of the cells that regulate your immune system live in your guts?

So if you are serious about your health, and I know you are because otherwise you wouldn't have read this far, you need to take a closer look at boosting your immune system, which we'll do with this diet.

## How do you get Candida?

If your immune system is weakened through prolonged illness, you are more likely to get a yeast infection. The contraceptive pill, diabetes and antibiotics are also well known contributing factors of Candida overgrowth. Is it contagious? No, it's not. So unless your partner has taken antibiotics and has a low immune system, he should be fine. You, on the other hand, can still re-infect yourself through your partner until your immune system is back to working on all cylinders.

For instance, if you feel run down and you are exposed to higher Candida levels (through kissing or sex), then you can get oral or vaginal thrush — a condition in which Candida accumulates on the lining of your mouth/ vagina. *So watch out.* A diet rich in fast food and sugar will also further promote Candida, as it is the ideal breeding ground for yeast. Constipation is also known to promote Candida growth.

## How do you prevent Candida?

Regular exercise can help to re-activate a sluggish digestive system, which in turn helps to prevent Candida. So as long as your immune system is strong, you eat a balanced diet and avoid taking antibiotics, you'll be fine. And don't start worrying about taking a contraceptive, please. It alone will not give you Candida. It is only a contributing factor.

You won't get Candida from just one factor. Inflammation is always an accumulative effect from lots of factors going wrong *for years*. This is where the Candida diet plan comes in handy. Once the Candida is under control, this diet will help you maintain a healthy balance, ensuring you never get Candida again.

## So what do you do when you suspect you have Candida?

First of all, determine the area of your body that may be exhibiting symptoms. Then, compare it to a list of typical Candida symptoms -- like the one on page 10.

If you are still unsure about the result, you can have a blood, urine and stool test done (a spit test is the least reliable test). But go through the list now -- it will give you a fairly good idea whether you've got it.

## Candida symptoms versus cold/ hay fever symptoms

It's usually quite hard to differentiate between a yeast infection and a cold or hay fever, as Candida symptoms are virtually the same. Yeast infections can make you feel equally as groggy.

## Signs of a simple yeast infection

If your immune system is healthy, you are likely to only experience a very localized infection of the skin or mucous membranes of your body. The most well-known type of Candida symptom in women is vaginal thrush.

Other common Candida symptoms include redness, itchiness and discomfort in the affected area.

Typically, infections are of the nose, sinuses, throat area right down to the stomach, digestive organs and genitals – oral and vaginal thrush being the most common type of infection. Chances are that if it's warm and moist, you can get a yeast infection in that part of your body. Sadly, by the time most people find out about their Candida infection, it has become systemic, virtually encompassing all the Candida symptoms mentioned below.

## Candida die-off symptoms

When your body manages to eliminate some Candida, it produces poisonous by-products that are seriously uncomfortable local disorders of a Candida infection. This is also called Candida die-off.

Review the helpful checklist on the next page to quickly assess if your problems might be Candida related.

## Self-Diagnosis Help -- Candida Symptoms Checklist:

- Cravings for sweet food and bread (yeast feeds on sugar)
- Mood swings, depression, increased heartbeat ore even palpitations and sudden anxiety attacks
- Candida interferes with hormones
- Feeling "woozy" after eating a lot of carbs (yeast produces alcohol)
- Feeling low and tired (particularly after a meal)
- Feeling bloated and/or gassy
- Constipation or diarrhea, IBS
- Skin infections, itchy skin, eczema, rashes and nail fungus
- Food allergies, hay fever
- Sinuses, lung and throat infections
- Urinary tract infections, thrush (Candidiasis), low libido, painful intercourse
- Joint pain, stiff joints
- Edema (e.g., swollen ankles)
- PMS
- Loss of memory, foggy thinking
- Thyroid problems, hair loss
- Insomnia
- Muscle twitching, cramps
- Numb or tingling feeling in fingers or toes
- Dry, irritable or infected eyes
- Sensitivity to smoke, perfume and damp, moldy environments

## What's your score? How many Candida symptoms do you have?

If you selected more than three boxes, there is a distinct chance that the symptoms you're experiencing might stem from a yeast infection.

To be certain, you can take a Candida test. Regardless of the outcome, though, I'd recommend you follow the Candida diet for a few weeks to see if it helps get rid of your symptoms.

If you selected one of the highlighted options, it looks like you already have a yeast infection. This can be sorted out very quickly.

If, however, you've selected more than six boxes, I'm afraid it's highly likely that your Candida symptoms are not coincidence but signs of a systemic yeast infection. You can treat this naturally, too, so don't worry. It just requires a bit more of a systematic approach and will take a bit longer.

The diet outlined in this book will help get your symptoms under control and get your health back. Apart from menu suggestions of what you can eat, you'll also find lots of tips and natural remedies for any symptoms you might have.

## My Candida Story

Let me set the stage for you.

I like to think that I had a reasonably normal lifestyle growing up. Granted, there were a few ups and downs... but then who doesn't have those?!

Yes, looking back now I can see that I had a weak immune system. I had a semi-constant congested nose and sore throat -- surely not helped from skipping breakfast, watching late night TV or reading my fantasy books. But then that's normal, right?!

Hell, when I was a teenager, I lived for the weekend. My life consisted of even more late nights, alcohol, instant pasta and pizza. But come on people -- that's just what teenagers do, RIGHT?!!

Maybe the tipping point for me was doing a seven-year law degree. That, my friends, is a ton of pressure balanced only by a ton of comfort food.

Let's not dwell on this too much, but here's a few symptoms I was experiencing:

- Emotions up and down.
- My periods were very bleedy and crampy.
- I constantly felt touchy and bloated.
- Sex was a disaster with intercourse being very painful.
- Yep, I was a bundle of joy! Both on the inside and out.

- So by the time I was in my twenties, I was experiencing excruciating lower belly ache. But that's what painkillers are for, right?

- My gynecologist kept prescribing me different antibiotics and told me to drink cranberry juice. And my urologist? Well, my urologist saw it fit to insert a 20 cm long ice cold tube with a camera into my bladder, leave me waiting half naked with spread legs in his room while assistants were coming and going, only to tell me... *that I was imagining my illness!!*

After that, I decided to see a specialist. My sneezing fits, coughing and general lack of well-being were beyond the norm... even for me! He injected 30 different substances under my skin to evaluate any potential allergies. Welcome to HELL!

My entire arm swelled to the size of something very big, I felt instantly sick and light-headed and I had the most INTENSE ITCH EVER! All to which the specialist smiled, handed me a salve and a list of all the things I showed a response to, and sent me on my way.

Mold and dust mites, by the way. Those things to me were like Kryptonite to Superman!

So let's have a quick recap.

- I'm a complete mess.
- I have my final exam coming up for my seven-year law degree.
- I'm suffering from irrational anxiety and panic attacks.
- I'm hyper, nervous, losing weight, my eyes are always irritable

- and.... *My hair is getting thinner*?!! What the *@$*?!
- But hey-ho! I'm just nervous because of my exams, right?!

Finally, I saw another doctor after severe sleep deprivation. He prescribed me tranquilizers and took a blood test. My blood test came back and, wait for it ladies and gentlemen.... my thyroid hormone levels were 20 times that of a normal person. You could say that I was very, *very ill!*

For the next 2.5 years, I took hardcore thyroid and beta blockers. That reduced my discomfort to a manageable level of horror, but still not desirable. Not only that, I started displaying a new set of symptoms -- super sensitive dry skin.

It was like I was living in a "whack-a-mole" game. Hit one of the critters on the head and another two pop up somewhere else. That's right, folks; my prolonged stress, existential anxieties, disturbed sleep and a change in diet had joined forces and called into existence a new breed of terror -- *ECZEMA!*

But don't worry. As any doctor will tell you, eczema is fully treatable. Just slap on a bit of steroid cream and you'll be right as rain. What they don't tell you though is that steroids will not remove the problem. Think of it like painting over a damp and mouldy wall. Your paint job is screwed from the start -- you need to fix the problem first.

Well, one thing led to another and I started researching on the Web for other solutions. And I discovered that sugar is to blame for all this evil. So I went on a hardcore detox, followed by a refined sugar-free diet. But like all newly enlightened health junkies, I threw myself into this whole new world of "healthy" eating without actually knowing what I was doing.

I started taking olive leaf capsules because I had read that they boost the immune system. I drank gallons of fresh fruit juice and eagerly sweetened my tea with Manuka honey because I had learned that cane sugar is bad for you and honey is a natural healer.

I snacked on plenty of mixed cereals with dried fruit and oats –
so much better for you than cakes and sweets, right?

Easy mistake to make, especially considering the homeopath and
naturopath I had consulted with for advice in my desperation --
being covered in an intensely itchy, scaly skin condition from head
to toe does make you a little freaky at times, you know –
had assured me that my diet was very wholesome and good! So
why should I worry?

But the thing is, deep down in your heart of hearts you know when
things aren't doing you any good. You feel it. You might not
understand it. But you know you can't carry on the way you used
to. Just like you yourself have reached that point now where you
know that you are stuck. You are not getting better by doing what
you are currently doing. Fact.

Basically, by consuming all those "natural" sugars, I was feeding
the Candida big time. And by taking high doses of olive leaf
tablets, I was killing masses of Candida every day. So without
realizing it, I was creating an overload of "waste products" in my
blood stream that my poor liver couldn't process and my body --
ever so resourceful -- tried to eliminate all the toxins through my
skin. Hence the severe eczema flare ups.

I'm not going to lie to you. It took me three years to get fully well
again. Years of trial and error. Three years' worth of anti-Candida
dieting. Time spent trying to find nourishing recipes and testing
what remedies work. It was the cooking and baking in search of
palatable recipes that kept me sane in those dark times.

Every day of those three years, I wrote a food and treatment diary
to record my progress. I recommend you do the same.

Now, I want to share my findings with you so that your recovery is
as quick and painless as possible. I've put together this guide with
tips and recipes to get you started. Hopefully, it will answer all the
questions you have. I am still following a sugar-free, mostly
gluten-free diet, and not just to avoid a relapse.

I do it because I have actually grown to like this lifestyle and way of eating. There are a lot of wonderfully tasty dishes out there for you, once you start looking and experimenting. When I'm with family or friends, I can happily eat "the wrong foods" like chocolate or cake. But I make sure I balance it out the next day.

I know you are probably worried now that you can't ever enjoy pizza or the odd glass of wine again. And that's perfectly normal. I thought the same thing when I started the diet. But I can tell you that you will be able to eat all the foods again that you used to love. You really will! Just not right now and not all the time. Chances are, you won't even want to as your taste buds and your habits change. *(I know you don't believe me yet and that's ok!)*

The main thing is that by adopting a healthy diet, you are setting the foundation for looking great and feeling better than you have in years!

If you have more questions on your mind, head on over to my blog at www.candidadietplan.com. I'm constantly adding new recipes and info about Candida and healthy eating in general. And I thoroughly enjoy conversation with like-minded health warriors. I'd love for you to connect with me personally so I can follow your journey to health.

## Curing Candida is a Four Step Process:

### 1. Fast/Candida Cleanse

**1-7 days with the option to continue doing this once a week/month as part of your health routine**

Only drink veggie juices and broth, in conjunction with colonics. This is to flush your system inside and out, killing Candida and streamlining your digestion.

### 2.  Strict Diet - 2 weeks with no carbs
Here you avoid allergens and foods that feed Candida.

That means no sugar, no fruit, no yeast, no bread… and a whole host of other foods and drinks you're not allowed that you'd normally have. Now you start taking antifungals to kill more Candida. I'll give you a list of highly effective options, and tell you when to take them and when to start with probiotics.

While you follow the diet, you remove layer upon layer of health issues. So depending on how many things are wrong with you, it takes a longer time.

Oftentimes, it's not the actual Candida symptoms that are the problem but the blockages and secondary health issues that result from the overgrowth. You might have developed a gluten or dairy intolerance or you might have red angry inflammations in your body that flare up when you eat meat.

To pinpoint exactly what doesn't agree with you, it's helpful to write down what you're eating and how you are feeling in a food diary. A few keywords will do, which will enable you to back-trace what might have upset you as sometimes reactions can appear days later. Generally, once you have followed a clean diet for a few months, you'll notice that you can tolerate more foods that would previously have caused a reaction.

### 3. Maintenance Diet

**4 weeks+ where you can now eat small amounts of root and starchy vegetables and grains, and start taking probiotics to fill the gaps that the Candida has left.**

Time to eat some cereals or yeast-free breads again, yippee. You are sure going to love this. Millet, beans, root vegetables, quinoa, buckwheat… anything goes as long as it is introduced gradually and you carefully determine if you are really ready for it.

If you display more symptoms after eating it (regardless how happy it made you to eat it!), you should go back to a mostly "Stage 2: strict diet" type diet until your immune system is stronger.

During this phase, you should still not eat anything with sugar, agave or fruit in it. You'll be taking antifungals until you are free from symptoms. And you'll be taking probiotics at least until the end of Stage 4.

**Stage 3 should really be split into two parts:**

The initial 4-6 weeks of dieting, taking antifungals and figuring out what foods might not agree with you, as well as healing one after the other health issue in your body.

The second part then consists of repeating meals that agree with you and taking probiotic supplements to gradually rebuild and strengthen your immune system.

Generally, what makes you ill is not so much the Candida itself, it's all the other health issues it allowed to happen. So by simply getting the Candida levels down, you'll still feel pretty horrendous. And your immune system could not support itself. Therefore, you'd get ill again very soon.

That's why it is essential that you get the number of friendly beneficial microorganisms up that build the basis of your immune system and help with the digestion of food. For that, you need to take in HIGH amounts of probiotics and foods that they can feed on, like vegetables.

You'll also need to avoid anything that undermines your immune system. Most Candida diets put all the emphasis on a sugar-free diet but fail to mention how stress, lack of movement, sleep deprivation, unhappiness, an unhealthy environment and gluten intolerance or leaky gut can postpone or prevent people's permanent recovery.

**4. Transition to Normal Eating - 1 year**

Even when your symptoms have disappeared, you have to carry on with the diet. Slowly introduce some fruit into your diet, then bread low in yeast (e.g., pitta), then cheese and cow's milk.

When you can tolerate all of those -- congratulations, you have your life back! It is recommended to carry on with the diet on the maintenance level (Stage 3) with the occasional "off day" to avoid any relapse.

During Stage 4, your immune system is not yet strong enough to control a potential Candida overgrowth on its own. It only keeps it at a certain level. A traumatic event, a mega sugar binge or a period of stress can easily cause a relapse, so it's best to protect what you've worked so hard for. You can still go all out on special occasions, birthdays and such. Think fruit, cheese, booze, cake, ice cream… just don't make it the rule.

**How long will it take you to recover?**

**It usually takes a month of clean eating for every year you have had Candida problems.**

So if you have had Candida for the past 12 years, it would take you about a year to get fully well again. But it always depends on how ill you are to begin with.

- Do you have any other illnesses?
- Are you under a lot of stress?
- Are you prepared to follow the diet very strictly or are you planning on continuing to eat certain fruit and cereals or chocolate and the odd glass wine?
- Are you mineral deficient?
- Are you suffering from heavy metal poisoning?
- Are you living in an old house that has a mold problem?
- Do you have food allergies?
- How active are you?
- How happy are you? Sadness severely undermines your immune system and really slows down your recovery.

There are so many factors that play into this.
But generally, if you are consistently working on getting rid of Candida, then *it should take you a month for every year you've had it*.

If you only have a mild yeast infection, then you should be right as rain in about a month.

If you've had recurring yeast infections, it will take you a little longer. But you'll definitely feel a lot better in just a few weeks. You really will. And you'll learn valuable insights about your body and health tips in general that will stand you in good stride for the rest of your life.

# CHAPTER TWO

## STAGE ONE OF THE DIET – CLEANSE (2 DAYS RECOMMENDED)

**Why do you need to fast?**

It's simple. If you don't feel in tip-top shape, it's a sign that your body is struggling with something.

Helping your body detox and letting go of what is no longer needed is one of the best ways to *boost your immune system and feel on top of things again!* Your body does a lot of its healing and restoration work at night when you are asleep or resting deeply. Now -- how well do you sleep? I think we both know the answer -- not as well as you used to. Not as long as you used to. Forget about a power nap during the day – there's no time for that! And when was the last time you got out of bed in the morning with a spring in your step and a song on your lips?!

So if your body is having a hard time keeping up with all the internal shenanigans, why not make it easy and *focus the energy that you normally spend on getting, preparing, eating and digesting food onto healing instead*? Don't forget that by simply doing a Candida cleanse, you can *get rid of a fair share of Candida in one fell swoop*. If you flush your kidneys and liver before starting the diet, you'll feel much better for it!

## Who should NOT do a fast?

If you are **underweight or fragile due to prolonged illness or old age a fast is not a good idea**, at least not without supervision from a doctor.

The same applies **when you are pregnant or breast feeding**. During those times you need the extra energy from the food, including carbs. I recommend you eat lots of veggies, brown rice, good oils and fish. You can still tackle the diet once your baby doesn't need to be breast fed and you've had a chance to breathe.

## What you need to do:

## 1. Take the strain off your digestive system

Most people think the idea of a fast is to "not eat and basically starve yourself." That couldn't be further from the truth. You need nourishment – whether you fast or not, and especially when you are already ill like you are now. So please don't approach Stage 1 by just cutting out the foods that you normally eat. You need nutrients -- plenty of them and in an easily digestible form (i.e., drinks and soups)!

So make sure that you take in plenty of mineral rich vegetable or bone broth. To understand how your digestive system works and what foods agree with what I recommend reading "Dr. Ali's Nutrition Bible" - explained in simple terms with healthy recipes and health tips in general - very good.

## 2. Relax
Focus your energy on healing and on what is important to you. Take stock: *Do you spend enough time doing the things you love? With the people you care about?*

## 3. Aid your body's elimination process
With these simple tricks, you can aid the detoxification even further:

- Drink 3 liters or more to flush out toxins
- Exercise to pump oxygen around your body
- Massage to get your lymph system working
- Sauna and steam baths help you sweat out toxins and build up your resistance to infections
- Body brushing improves circulation
- Flush out toxins with enemas and colonics

And on that note, I came across an eBook called *"How And When To Be Your Own Doctor"* by Dr. Isabelle A. Moser with Steve Solomon. It's freely available as far as I know -- just google it. Chapter 4 gives interesting advice about diy colon cleansing. Seeing as the colon is the number 1 area where Candida loves to reside, it helps to get clued up on this territory that is rarely spoken about. Learning how to administer colonic enemas yourself at home saves you on expensive colonic treatments in the long term. Professional colonics are recommended for newbies though — for ease of use and because they are much more effective.

**So, here's what you do: For 48-hour drink only detox teas and broth -- you can easily slip that in over a weekend. Nothing too extreme!**

But before you do that I highly recommend eating very light meals for 3-5 days to ease yourself into the fast. Cooked brown rice, fish, steamed vegetables, soups and celery with hummus are fabulous foods for the transition. Of course, you can extend the fasting period itself to 7 days instead of 48 hours if you think you can fit that in. That's what I did the first time round. Be prepared to feel physically weak and emotionally low though. So working and exercising are not possible without risking exertion and ultimately health complications (happened to me!).

You can see the exact detox protocol I followed on my blog. If you don't know where to start or you're simply curious what my detox protocol looked like then visit http://candidadietplan.com/candida-cleanse/

## What to eat/ What not to eat

To eat? The cheek of it! You are not really meant to eat
ANYTHING! If you really can't go without food, opt for steamed
vegetables and go straight to Stage 2. But really, what have you got
to lose? Just try the fast for a day!

## Drinks you can have during your fast (as much as you want):

- Freshly brewed ginger tea
- Nettle and mullein tea
- Dandelion tea
- Filtered water
- Water with apple cider vinegar (ACV)
- Chamomile tea
- Green goodness juice
- Fasting or detox tea
- Hot veggie and bone broth

## Green Goodness Juice

- 1 handful fresh spinach and watercress leaves
- 1 handful basil, parsley or coriander (cilantro)
- half a large organic cucumber
- 1-2 stalks celery
- juice of 1 small lemon or lime
- 1 chopped clove garlic
- 1/2 teaspoon spirulina powder (or chlorella/ barley grass)

Mix and drink as quickly as possible - before the herb taste hits
you!

## Tomato Basil Pick Me Up Juice

- 6 ripe tomatoes on the vine
- 1 handful fresh basil leaves
- a sprinkle salt and freshly ground black pepper
- a sprinkle of garlic granules

Wash, chop, whizz -- enjoy! This snack is sweet and pleasant; very different from the green goodness juice!

**Snacks:**

- Avocado, chilled cucumber slices
- ½ cup cooked brown rice with coconut oil
- hot cup of veggie broth

Make a hearty veggie broth and bone broth. Alongside the fasting tea and the odd green juice, this will keep you going.

You know as well as I do -- you can't go through an entire weekend, let alone a week, without eating ANYTHING! Have some avocados and chilled cucumber slices handy to snack on when you are starving.

Or as a last resort, you could nibble on a bit of cooked brown rice with coconut oil. Make sure you chew it well and eat it re-a-l-l-y slowly. Aim for 1-2 tablespoons, a small bowl at the most. Yes, rice contains carbs, but it is nutrient rich, easy to digest and your body needs some energy to focus properly and handle any stress or activity. Candida is still being killed as you are not actively feeding the yeast, so don't worry about that if you eat it only once.

**What NOT to eat:**

What you should not have is **meat, cereal, oats, bread or dairy** -- that said, out of all of those things, dairy is the lesser of the evils. But just see if you can wait with eating yoghurt until the strict diet. That would be cool. Try not to get stressed out about the meals and the preparation though. Stress is just as bad as eating sugar!

**Are there any side effects when embarking on a Candida cleanse?**

Unfortunately, there might be. And I don't mean your tummy rumbling sounds out of hunger!

If you kick start your metabolism with the Candida cleanse, it is possible that more Candida gets killed than your liver can break down -- and you'll feel ill because of all the Candida by-products in your system (i.e., acetylaldahyde and methane gas).

**This is called Candida die-off. Here's what you can do about it:**

You can avoid harsh die-off symptoms by taking things slowly and easing yourself into the fast while carefully monitoring your body's response. Plus, you can take herbs, vitamins and minerals that aid your liver's ability to break down toxins.

So even if you feel ill, you can make yourself feel better again quickly. For instance, drinking dandelion and burdock tea really helps, as does milk thistle tincture and resting a lot. Quickly take stock of where in your body you have discomfort. How does this compare with your symptoms assessment before you started the fast? (see symptoms checklist in Chapter 1).

**How do you know whether your symptoms are a good sign from the die-off or new additional symptoms?**

I know from my own experience that it can be very hard to differentiate between symptoms that are caused by Candida being killed off and new Candida symptoms, which indicate a relapse or standstill of the treatment. I have put together this checklist to help you analyze what may be going wrong so you can quickly get back on track.

**1. Symptom Check**
How are you feeling? Are there any new signs of Candida?

**2. Number of Symptoms**
Where exactly are the symptoms? Do they appear in one or several parts of your body? (Say first you feel it in your tummy, then your skin starts itching, then your eyes are irritable all within 40 minutes from taking antifungals -- this is an indicator that it's a die-off reaction).

### 3. History
Have you had this before?

### 4. Diet Sins
Have you eaten anything that isn't allowed on the Candida diet? (If your answer is yes, chances are it is likely to be a sign of a yeast overgrowth, which can show up 1 or 2 days after you've eaten the suspect food.) Have you perhaps eaten something that might have caused an allergic response like a food intolerance? Typical culprits are wheat, nuts, eggs and milk.

### Top Tip: Start a Food Diary!
Just record what you ate and whether your symptoms have worsened. Do this once a day or once a week, either in a note pad or online. You'll soon start to see patterns.

### 5. Higher Dose of Antifungals
Have you taken a higher dose of antifungals? (If yes, this indicates your symptoms could be die-off reactions. Bear in mind that even natural antifungals like garlic or coconut oil and even probiotic yoghurt can cause strong reactions that look just like Candida symptoms.)

### 6. Stress Factors
Were you stressed?

### 7. Weather
Was it raining outside? (More mold spores in the air means more Candida.)

### 8. Lack of Sleep
Did you sleep badly? (Your body can only heal when you get rest.)

### 9. Lack of Exercise
Were you sitting all day and had no movement or exercise?

**Get fresh air and get your heart pumping!** A walk in the morning and 60 star jumps in the afternoon is the minimum you should aim for if you want to get rid of the infections faster!

I'd keep the star jumps to the diet phase though - we don't want you to faint during your fast. A walk is just fine during those days!

Candida doesn't need oxygen but your healthy cells do, otherwise they cannot fight Candida off. So make sure you're working up a sweat in the gym or dancing to your favorite song at home.

You want to flush the baddies out of your system and out from every little corner. *If you keep moving, your body has a better chance of transporting all the Candida by-products out of your body via the lymph system.*

This system is only working when you're moving. If you're just sitting, the veins in your legs have real trouble transporting old blood back to your heart to replace it.

**TOP TIP: Help your body. Become active. Get some fresh air. Breathe deeply.**

### 10. Lifestyle
If you did do some exercise, was it exhausting or quite late in the day? Physically strenuous exercise leads to lactic acid in your muscles (i.e., muscle ache). Try massaging this away afterwards or body brushing to alleviate the already existing symptoms from the Candida toxins that are stored in your muscle tissues and joints.

Exercise also creates more dead Candida in your bloodstream. If you go to the gym in the evening, there might still be an overload of toxins in your system overnight as your body shuts down for the night. This might lead to things like a blocked nose when you wake up the next morning. It's best to exercise early and massage your legs or put them up high to encourage lymph drainage.

### 11. Lack of Oxygen
Were you in a stuffy environment and had no fresh air all day?

### 12. Bad Mood
Were you worried or unhappy?
Stress creates tension and an acidic cell environment that inhibits

healing and fosters Candida symptoms. But the more you try not to be stressed, the more hectic you'll get. Learn to direct your thoughts to something that creates a warm feeling in your belly, makes you feel happy or at least safe.

If you are stuck in a negativity loop or simply feeling rough, following a guided meditation is best. This will give your subconscious mind breathing space to kick-start your healing. There are some fantastic short guided meditations available to download on iTunes to get you started. A lot of them are free.

**TOP TIP: Listen to a Guided Meditation with Music!**

There is one particular meditation that I recommend you try. It is the first one I ever listened to and it's brilliant.

It really takes your mind of things. It's from Meditation Oasis and it's called "Deep Relaxation." It lasts for 20-25 minutes, and it's just a friendly female voice talking to you with soft music in the background. Not what you'd expect if you hear the word "meditation."

And when you try things like exercise or meditation -- always remember that the benefits might not be noticeable straight away. Don't let that dishearten you. Only after regular relaxation/meditation will you generally notice a relief in your symptoms.

If you answered "yes" to one or multiple of the questions above, chances are your symptoms are a bit more than just die-off. Or perhaps you just created an extra burden for your body to heal the existing symptoms. So your progress with the Candida diet is stagnating. Everyone goes through periods of stress or occasions where you overindulge on foods that promote Candida.

You've just got to realize that. And when you notice that you have reached a plateau where you feel especially run down and panicky, just give yourself a rest.

If you do encounter strong die-off symptoms, focus on how you can make it better from that moment on. Try not to analyze what you might have done wrong too much. Instead, view this incident as a positive sign that your body is booting up your immune system.

You only need to work on fine-tuning it. Believe me, not giving into thinking that "it will never heal" and learning to let go is the hardest thing to do. I've slowed my own recovery down myself -- involuntarily -- because I was so stressed with my job and even when I was at home, I felt I was running out of time. It was only after I learned to manage my stress levels better that I managed to get my Candida under control.

If you feel you don't have the time to do relaxing things, challenge your beliefs. What is the worst thing that can happen if you stopped for 30 minutes to lie down with closed eyes listening to calming music instead of rushing around? It only takes a few more positive healthy choices in your life to tilt the scales and help you heal. If I can heal, so can you -- I can assure you of that! If going to festivals, changing jobs and eating the odd slice of gateaux cake didn't permanently sabotage the recovery from Candida for me, it can't do for you either – regardless of how hopeless you might feel right now.

Remind yourself when you hit rock bottom that you cannot think clearly when you have an acute Candida infection -- it really plays havoc with your emotions. So trying to make sense of it all in that situation is bound to fail. Just keep working at it a day at a time and you will combat Candida once and for all.

## Recap of Stage 1: Fasting cleanses your body

*You'll heal faster* when you do a 2-7 day cleanse before starting the diet. Veggie juice and broth recipes are the best way to tide you over during that time.

In this chapter, you've found answers to lots of cleanse related questions. You've learned that you can experience an onset of initial discomforts called *die-off symptoms,* found out how to identify them and also *how to make yourself feel better.*

**Top Tip:** If you're on Facebook , join the supplementary Candida Diet Facebook Group "Detox Buddies" at https://www.facebook.com/groups/461481663913951/ for free moral support on this journey.

# CHAPTER THREE

## STAGE TWO - 2 WEEKS STRICT DIET & REMEDIES

**Why you need to stick to a strict diet**

The idea of this phase is to *stop feeding Candida* and to *take remedies to kill it*. Not only that but also to *reverse the food allergies or grain sensitivities* that you might have developed from having Candida and eating the wrong foods. These are generally only temporary because your immune system is just a bit over-reactive. But that's why you're not allowed to eat any cereals, bread or pasta (i.e., all grains) in Stage 2 and why the diet is so strict.

**What you need to do:**

You follow a strict sugar-free diet for 2 weeks. During that time, you only eat foods that are allowed on the Candida diet. The idea is to eat as healthily as possible and to improve your digestion. You also need to take remedies to kill Candida and to heal the secondary health issues it has caused.

**Here are some useful tips for improved digestion and a speedy recovery:**

- Drink fresh ginger tea
- Take a good multivitamin and mineral complex
- Take spirulina/chlorella for extra energy
- Drink apple cider vinegar (ACV)
- Aim to eat a light dinner no later than 6 p.m. and stay away from greasy food
- Eat healthy portions (i.e., don't have seconds, have a big portion of veg)
- Use good fats like coconut oil
- Add spices and herbs for cooking and as natural remedies
- Go for a quick walk morning and evening
- Drink loose nettle/dandelion tea and mint/chamomile tea
- Grill, steam or bake your food instead of frying it
- Take a power nap after lunch and aim to be in bed by 10.30 p.m.
- Make a point of doing something relaxing and solely enjoyable more often

Remember, changing your eating habits is a big step. But if you strive to live just a little bit healthier every week, you'll be amazed what you can achieve! Stay with it. You've made a fantastic start, and you're not alone!

Now before I show you what remedies you can take, let's take a look how you can simplify your diet and lifestyle during the 2 weeks of strict diet (Stage 2). In other words, what can you eat?

**What to eat  -  Food List for Stage 2**

Basically, you can enjoy all the drinks from Stage 1 here, too. And you can pretty much enjoy as many of the foods listed here as you like, as they are incredibly good for you and promote your healing.

It might not seem like it but there are actually delicious foods that you are allowed to eat!

You're probably thinking right now that you won't be able to eat ANYTHING! Am I right?!

Easy tiger, you'll be fine.

Also, remember that there are many different variations of Candida diets out there. They all allow you slightly different foods to eat. Don't let that confuse you. Just like there are conflicting opinions in your family about what tastes nice and what's good for you, there are just as many different camps amongst Candida sufferers who have their very own ideas of what helped them and what didn't. Go with common sense and decide whether it fits your taste buds and lifestyle.

If you are unsure about including a certain food item that's not on this list, then just email me and ask me! Don't be shy.

**Protein-rich foods that you can eat**

- Eggs
- Fish (fresh, frozen and tinned)
- Poultry (preferably fresh and organic)
- Bacon (unsmoked)

**Why I also include bacon on my Candida diet food list:**

Cured meat is not healthy, don't get me wrong. I'm not telling you this is the optimum diet. All I'm saying is if you are used to eating a lot of hams and meats like I am (hey, I come from Sauerkraut land -- I had no choice), then you can still eat it occasionally.

I tend to sprinkle some grilled bacon over cauliflower soup or omelette twice a week, and I'm prepared to live with that vice as I really enjoy it and I'm sticking to the Candida diet in every other respect.

## Veg

- Avocado
- Cucumbers, courgettes (zucchinis), celery
- Green & leafy vegetables (e.g., kale, spring greens/ collard, chard, spinach, watercress, French beans, broccoli, handful of peas)
- Tomatoes, bell peppers, aubergine (eggplant)
- Salad (avoid the mixed pre-packed variety)
- Onions, leek, garlic
- Artichoke, fennel, asparagus
- Chickpeas (they are actually a vegetable and not a bean, believe it or not)
- Fresh herbs (basil, coriander, mint, lemon balm)
- Sea vegetables/algae (e.g., nori, wakame, etc.)

## Oils

- Coconut oil
- Olive oil
- Flax/ Linseed oil (not for cooking)

## Stock & Salad Sauces, Seasoning and Spices

- Yeast-free stock cubes and homemade bone broth
- Coconut aminos
- Bragg's seasoning (non-fermented soya sauce)
- Organic tomato paste (as long as it contains no citric acid)
- Low salt or sea salt, freshly ground black pepper, turmeric, cayenne pepper, ginger spice, garlic, thyme
- Apple cider vinegar, olive oil and lemon juice
- Cinnamon, vanilla

## Menu Suggestions for Stage 2:

vegetable omelette, vegetable soup, chicken soup, steamed vegetables and fish, grilled chicken breast, stir-fry

## Best Snack:

- Avocado, green smoothie, hummus and celery sticks
  (preferably make your own hummus or buy organic)
- As a weekend treat:

your favorite toasted yeast free bread with almond butter, and in terms of baked treat an unsweetened coconut muffin is your safest bet but best to wait until stage 3

## Best Baking Ingredients

- Ground almonds/almond flour, stevia (no sweetener is best)
- Coconut flour, desiccated coconut, flax seeds
- Rice milk (best diluted)/unsweetened almond milk/coconut
  milk/semi skimmed goat's milk

## Superfoods and Protein Powder for Extra Energy

- Chlorella, spirulina, maca, barley grass, hemp seeds
- In terms of protein powder, go for hemp or pea protein

## Allowed Only Once or Twice per Week

- Cooked brown rice (small bowl full with coconut oil and
  cinnamon, chewed slowly)
- Probiotic yoghurt (small tub)
- Handful of sunflower seeds or pumpkin seeds
- Handful of nuts (preferably freshly cracked; almonds are best)

## Food Ideas for Vegans

- Increase the intake of dark green vegetables and sea
  vegetables like nori and wakame; they are higher in protein.
  You can then add lightly roasted sunflower and/or sesame
  seeds to give it a bit more substance.
- Sprinkle lots of ground flax seeds or de-shelled hemp seeds
  over your meals.
- Small amounts of tofu are okay.

- Chickpeas would also make a great addition for vegans on a Candida diet. Before breakfast, you could have a spirulina drink, which is a real vitamin, mineral and protein powerhouse.
- Perhaps you might want to try a green vegetable juice or green smoothie -- you could add a bit of pea or hemp protein powder to fill you up for longer and add extra nutrients.
- Rice milk, coconut milk and almond milk are great milk alternatives and you could have a small amount of unsweetened soya yoghurt if you like.

Hang in there -- in Stage 3, you can have more variety including quinoa.


## List of Hot Drinks allowed on our Yeast-free Diet

- Green tea
- Chamomile, peppermint, dandelion, lemon balm and lemon verbena tea (calms nerves and aids digestion)

- Ginger tea (double thumb size piece of ginger chopped and boiled in 1 liter+ of water)
- Hot water (cooking the water for 20 minutes or longer makes it alkaline, very good for you)
- Nettle mullein tea (detoxifying, combats cold symptoms, buy as loose tea and mix yourself)
- Hot lemon
- Dandelion root coffee (not the granules as they contain sugar)
- Pau d'Arco tea


## List of Cold Drinks You Can Have

- Filtered water (lots of it!)
- Almond milk and occasionally soya milk if you like
- Small amounts of rice milk (I diluted mine with water for oatmeal porridge)

- Apple cider vinegar drink (2 teaspoons of cloudy ACV diluted in a glass of water -- drink upon awakening and before/with every meal, if you can stomach it. Some people are sensitive and need to heal those areas first.)
- Ice cold sparkling water with fresh lemon juice
- Green juice (glass of water with 1/2 teaspoon of chlorella powder, a hint of spirulina and the optional juice from half a lemon)
- Green smoothie (for instance, combine celery, cucumber, chilled coconut milk, cinnamon or vanilla, barley grass powder and ground linseeds/flax)
- Homemade lemonade with lime, stevia and lemon balm (this is a tip from my lovely reader, Sabine)
- Aim to drink at least 2-3 liters of these healthy beverages to help your body flush out Candida

As you move along with the diet, you'll be allowed more and more tasty foods. You'll see that even the list *"what you can eat"* in Stage 3 includes lots of nice things to look forward to –

Like pancakes and bread. So, don't be sad. It's only 2 weeks that you'll have to stick to this list -- that'll be gone in no time! And before you know it, the Candida diet is over and you can enjoy a big cup of cafe latte or hot chocolate again. It's worth fighting for.

**P.S.: Fancy some recipes for this stage of the diet? Check out my blog** at http://candidadietplan.com/best-candida-diet-recipes/. It's free!

**Here's a list of all foods to avoid if you follow the Candida diet:**

The foods you should avoid either contain sugar, which is not allowed, or they contain fermented produce, which you should step away from too if you want to succeed with this diet.

Another reason why the food mentioned here is not recommended for Candida sufferers is that it creates an acidic environment that promotes inflammations.

You guessed it -- all the usual goodies that taste sweet and scrumptious are off the books right now. What a shame!

## Sweet Foods

- Sugar, honey, agave, coconut sugar
- Fresh and dried fruit, jam
- Chocolate, carob and sweets (Chocolate disrupts your biorhythm and makes your blood sugar levels spike – even with stevia!)
- Cakes, biscuits and other sweet bakery treats
- Any flour (or pasta) -- the body breaks it down into sugar

- Mushy starchy/sweet vegetables (e.g., potato mash, beetroot, sweet potatoes, parsnips – not completely forbidden but better not eaten before Stage 3 of the Candida diet as they provide quick release energy for the yeast)

- Muesli with dried fruit -- hard to digest and full of sugar
- Porridge or any packaged cereal (e.g., wheat flakes, bran, rice crispies)

## Fermented or Containing Additives

- Cheese
- Mushrooms (watch out for Quorn, which is made from fungus)
- Bread and bakery products
- Battered food including scotch eggs, fish or sausages
- Anything containing fermented food like soya sauce and vinegar (with the exception of apple cider vinegar)
- Stock cubes with yeast

## Foods that are Difficult to Digest

- Canned foods with citric acid (e.g. tomatoes -- or coconut milk if half of the content is guar gum or other additives -- go for organic just water added)

- Hot spicy sauces (these kill all bacteria in your gut, even the good ones, also highly acidic and oily foods in particular are difficult to digest)
- Deep fried food (many free radicals and vitamin depleting)
- Red meats (it sits in your intestines for a long, long time as it is so hard to break down ---the longer it sits, the more chance to putrefy and that is what we're desperately trying to avoid here as you need as much energy as possible to fight Candida)

**Foods that Cause an Allergic Response**

- Oats/wheat -- Many people have an intolerance to these grains. I would have never admitted it myself because I loved eating this convenience food too much. Not to mention bagels and cheesy toasted sandwiches! That aside, every cereal packet under the sun has added sugar in one form or another (disguised as fructose, malt, dextrose, syrup)

- Nuts (unless freshly cracked; apparently, the shelled ones contain unseen mould)
- Sweetener -- makes your blood sugar levels spike, which encourages yeast growth

**Drinks that are Not Permitted on the Candida Diet**

- Coffee (stimulants make the body release sugar reserves into the blood stream as readily available energy; the dirty little scoundrels can even feed on that, if you can believe that)
- Alcohol, Lemonade, energy drinks, etc.
- Milk (contains milk sugars and is mucous producing)
- Fruit juices (even freshly squeezed!) and smoothies

**But at least you can have these snacks in Stage 2:**

The best snacks are generally leftovers from a meal you've had.

Chicken soup is a good choice, as is vegetable leftovers from the day before -- quickly re-heated and sprinkled with a bit of pumpkin seed oil, salt and pepper.

## Another quick snack option is a Veggie Sesame Stir-Fry:

Chop some leek, cabbage, courgette (zucchini), broccoli or other green veg. Then lightly fry it in coconut or sesame oil, sprinkle some sesame seeds and salt over it.

## Homemade Hummus

One can of chickpeas, juice of one small lemon, handful of freshly ground sesame seeds (or 2 tablespoons of tahini), one chopped garlic clove, ½ teaspoon salt, bit of water, olive oil -- mix and enjoy (this tastes often better the next day). Nibble with celery and bell pepper sticks.

**Almond Butter** (in moderation – you wouldn't eat 80 almonds in one go either, would you?! Nuts can cause indigestion)

## Chilled Cucumber Slices

I know, I've already recommended this in Stage 1.
But it's incredibly good for you (and not half as bad as it sounds).
Refreshing, calming and filling. Seriously!

## Simple Green Coconut Smoothie

- ⅓ can of coconut milk (with solids)
- dash of unsweetened almond milk
- Chlorella
- 1/2 organic cucumber
- sprinkle of cinnamon
- 2 heaped teaspoons desiccated coconut

Chop the cucumber into slices or cubes. Fill the blender with all the ingredients, including the cucumber, and blend until everything is smooth and creamy.

**P.S.: You have seen the massive recipes section on my blog, haven't you?!** It would be a shame if you missed those!

Go to http://candidadietplan.com/best-candida-diet-recipes/

**Why you need Antifungal Remedies:**

You stop feeding Candida by following a sugar-free diet, so you might think that it would wither and die. Unfortunately, that's not the case. Candida is a tenacious organism that can survive indefinitely in the most hostile environments.

No big surprise since its friendly base form's purpose is to decompose dead matter. So while you're dieting, some of the Candida retreats into a dormant spore-form. And the moment you eat normal again -- BAM -- your familiar health issues come back with a vengeance.

That's why you need to take remedies specifically for killing Candida. Now since I'm a big believer of treating your body naturally and holistically, you won't find me recommending you take synthetic or prescriptive antifungals.

I have yet to see these work long term. I have had far too many readers approach me at their wit's end after a Candida relapse after several doses of Diflucan or whatever meds doctors give you for a yeast infection. And think of all the side effects!

I've tried every natural antifungal under the sun and **what has worked best for me is Caprylic acid, olive leaf, grapefruit seed extract and oil of oregano.** That's why I'm only going to talk about these here. There are other effective antifungals on the market.

I've talked in a lot more detail about their benefits and side effects on my blog at http://candidadietplan.com/home-remedies/antifungal/
in case you want to delve deeper into this topic.
Now I cannot guarantee that you will respond equally well to

these. But there is a high probability as they have been successfully used by millions of people. Pick any two of these natural Candida remedies -- they're the only antifungals you'll ever need!

Most people see great results from eating pure *coconut oil.* **Oil of oregano and olive leaf extract** are perhaps THE most effective weapons in the fight against Candida, even in stubborn systemic cases *(highly effective for sinus infections and thrush).*

**Caprylic acid (derived from coconut oil),** in comparison, is a much gentler solution that predominantly targets the Candida in your gut as it also leaves more of your friendly bacteria intact. On the other hand, oil of oregano and olive leaf extract pretty much nuke everything! And if you have animals, perhaps your symptoms are caused by parasites. A very potent antifungal combination that addresses this issue is a tincture made from *wormwood, black walnut and cloves. Grapefruit seed extract* is the cheapest of the lot.

**Here's a list of useful foods and herbs that you can easily add to your diet too. They all have Candida killing and general immune system boosting properties:**

- Garlic
- Coconut oil
- Cloves
- Thyme
- Aloe vera
- Apple cider vinegar (ACV)
- Cinnamon
- Ginger
- Pau d'Arco and lemon balm tea

**One word of warning about garlic though:**

Be careful, as this really is a very pokey antifungal -- it actually can annihilate any friendly bacteria in your gut and cause sores in your mouth!

So it's bad news for any probiotics you might be taking. Try eating a tiny amount of garlic first to see how you react and even if it agrees with you, don't eat it every day.

And always take extra probiotics a few hours afterwards to replenish the "friendlies" in your gut. To keep it short and sweet, there really is no "one antifungal fits all."

You have to evaluate yourself based on how severe your symptoms are. Every single antifungal I've just mentioned here works a treat, so just pick one or two and go with it. It's also a good idea to rotate antifungals every week. But there is no right or wrong way -- every person is different.

And although you can follow a proven Candida protocol that exactly outlines what antifungal and when to take it, at the end of the day you will still have to fine-tune this system and adapt it to your very own requirements. It's a learning curve.

*The suggestions I make are not intended as treatment advice -- especially regarding the dosage guidelines. Please work with a specialist to put together a treatment plan that is right for you.*

## Antifungal Dosage Guidelines:

- **Coconut oil dosage:** Start with eating a teaspoon of coconut oil three times a day. Then gradually increase the amount until you can take 5 tablespoons without major die-off symptoms. If you can't imagine eating it straight, then Caprylic acid is the antifungal for you.

- **The Caprylic acid tabs** come in three different strengths, which makes them perfect for newbies as they can start with a lower dosage to avoid major die-off symptoms. Caprylic acid dosage: Start with the 250mg strength -- 1 capsule daily with a meal. Increase up to three times daily.

When you are able to handle this dosage, move to the 400mg starting with one again, continually adding one more until you are taking 3 capsules two times a day without new symptoms. Tackle the 680mg in the same fashion.

- **Grapefruit seed extract dosage:** Take 6-10 drops three times daily for 2-3 weeks at least 20 minutes before meals -- preferably 1 hour before.
  Start with once a day first and when tolerated well, take once more and so on.

  - **Olive leaf extract dosage:** Take 1 capsule 20 minutes before a meal once a day. When that agrees with you, slowly take 1 capsule more per day until you are taking 3 capsules two times per day.
  - You can drink the **Pau d'Arco** tea instead of ordinary tea in addition to your other antifungals.

**What antifungal worked best for me -- an example of long-term Candida management:**

For the first month, *I rotated grapefruit seed extract, wormwood, Pau d'Arco tea and olive leaf extract.*

Then I settled for olive leaf extract and took the capsules for over a year – *and it helped me, amongst others, get rid of my recurring sinus infections, foggy head, fatigue, depression and insomnia.* Unfortunately, the strong cleansing effect over-burdened my liver and I developed severe eczema all over my body.

Then I did another cleanse and started fresh again -- this time with *Caprylic acid, garlic and coconut oil.* This much gentler approach *allowed me to fully heal my skin inflammations and cravings, as well as most of the other remaining symptoms.* I kept that going for over half a year; however, prolonged use of large doses did not agree with me.

After that, I started taking much *higher strength probiotics and rotated olive leaf extract, oil of oregano and wormwood complex* weekly as needed when thrush re-occurred *(which was my last stubbornly remaining symptom)*.

This generally happened when I was under a lot of stress and I had eaten sugary foods.
Even now that my Candida levels are normal, I still include many food-related antifungals like *coconut oil, garlic, thyme and cinnamon* in my diet to discourage the yeast from overgrowing again.
I also still take probiotics twice daily.

But I have started eating more fermented foods in the hope that this will soon enable me to wean myself off the expensive probiotics.

**Recap: My treatment suggestion for you (especially beneficial for people with systemic Candida infections):**
*"Less is definitely more"* -- start with just the cleanse, putting particular emphasis on strengthening your liver, kidneys and immune system. No antifungal at this stage. If your die-off is not too savage, then opt for a gentle antifungal like Caprylic acid when starting the strict diet.

If you're suffering from die-off, keep off it until you feel better.
Two weeks later, add a high strength probiotic.
When you are no longer seeing results from the Caprylic acid, work your way up to oil of oregano or olive leaf extract. Rotate those until you are symptom free.

# Here are Eight Typical Candida Symptoms and Home Remedies to Cure Them:

- **Yoghurt to Cure Yeast Infections/ Vaginal Thrush -- the most common Candida symptom:**
Ladies: Insert a *tampon dipped in yoghurt* into your vagina for one to two hours at a time (up to twice a day until the thrush is gone).

Regular *douches/washes or sitz baths with diluted apple cider vinegar (ACV)* are also very beneficial. Depending on how long you have had Candida, your immune system might be very low so you might get symptoms in other parts of your body, too.
Men: I would presume that yoghurt and ACV washes work equally as well for men as for women. But it might be worth double-checking with a naturopath.

- **ACV wash and coconut moisturizer to combat "itch"**

A useful remedy is to *wash the area with an Apple cider vinegar solution* diluted with water and *use coconut oil or a lotion with tea tree oil as moisturizer.*

- **Oil pulling to heal oral thrush -- a furry white coating on your tongue**

Mix *almond oil (50 drops) with red thyme (1 drop), tea tree (1 drop) and cinnamon oil (1 drop)*. Keep this bottle in the fridge.

Whenever you feel you are coming down with something or when you have a white tongue, mix a few drops of this mixture with a *tablespoon of sunflower oil* and *swish it around in your mouth for a good 10-15 minutes before you brush your teeth or drink anything in the morning.* Spit it out and brush your teeth and tongue afterwards.

- **Colloidal silver and tea tree or shea butter for fungal skin infections**

You can treat fungal skin infections very effectively by spraying colloidal silver on it.
And by using coconut oil or a lotion with tea tree oil and shea butter to calm the sensitive skin.

- **Antibacterial drops to heal a sinus infection**

To heal a sinus infection mix, antibacterial drops with a combination of *sesame oil, mustard oil and double the amount of almond oil*. Place 1 drop into each nostril and sniff it up twice a day.

- **Gargle with sage to cure a sore throat**

If you develop a sore throat, you can quickly remedy it by gargling with a herbal tea called *sage tea*. Just buy the loose sage tea leaves and let them infuse in boiling water for 5 minutes. Let the tea cool down slightly before you gargle with it.

- **Clear up urinary tract infections with uva ursi**

Another fantastic loose herbal tea/tincture is *uva ursi*. This helps to clear up urinary tract infections, which is something that goes hand in hand with Candida. Even some popular commercial Candida remedies utilize this effect, such as "CandiGone."

- **Alleviate constipation with magnesium and lemon juice/vitamin C**

Constipation -- you can get a handle on with *lemon juice, magnesium supplements, lots of water, green tea, movement and by eating hummus, celery, cucumber, sauerkraut and cooked brown rice.* If you have stomach trouble with lemon juice, then try buffered vitamin C powder.

You can expect to have to treat your symptoms with natural remedies at least three times a day if they are severe or acute, for a minimum of 2 days. Persistent chronic Candida conditions often take weeks/months until all symptoms have disappeared. Don't expect to be healed over night. Crush your symptoms one by one, a day at a time.

For more information on Candida symptoms, remedies and common ailments in general, check out the Home Remedies section on my blog http://candidadietplan.com/home-remedies/.

## Recap of Stage 2: More Candida Gets Killed

Stage 2 of the diet is there so you *stop feeding Candida* and start *taking remedies to kill the Candida* off. The diet is also aimed at *bringing down the inflammation in your body* and to *start healing* all your symptoms.

# CHAPTER FOUR

## STAGE THREE - 4 WEEKS DIET AND PROBIOTICS

**Why you need to carry on with the diet**

As there's still Candida in your system, you'll need to carry on with a sugar-free diet, as well as continue taking antifungals. The idea of Stage 3 of the Candida diet is to *strengthen your immune system* while still *killing Candida.* To fill up the space that the dead Candida has left, you need to *start taking probiotics*.

**What you need to do:**

Keep following the diet. Just not quite as strictly as before. As your Candida overgrowth has gone down a bit, you can now *introduce small amounts of carbs and grains back into your diet* -- being it *root vegetables like potatoes, bread or cereal.*

Since you are taking antifungals that are bringing your Candida levels further down, there should be no danger of a relapse. The probiotics you are taking will help to make sure of that. As long as you still display symptoms after taking antifungal remedies, it makes sense to stay on the diet.

## What to eat - Food List for Stage 3

These are all the foods that I think you'll be able to eat without any problems. But they are just suggestions based on what agreed with me. You might be able to tolerate different foods, so feel free to adapt. In general though -- the stricter the diet, the quicker you'll recover.

### Protein-rich foods that you can eat

- Eggs
- Fish
- Poultry (preferably fresh and organic)
- Bacon (un-smoked; see Candida diet food list Stage 2 about why I think you can eat it)
- Feta or tofu (kefir, mozzarella and goat's cheese in bite-sized amounts only towards the end of the diet)
- Choose unpasteurized goat's or sheep's yoghurt over probiotic cow's milk yoghurt, (as this is easier to digest).

### Some clarification on why I think yoghurt and feta are okay to eat:

Some people don't allow any dairy on this diet. This is something you need to decide for yourself. There is no right or wrong way.

### Pros for including yoghurt and feta on the Candida diet food list:

The diet is hard enough as it stands. Yoghurt and feta are great sources of protein and as such, when you combine them with a small amount of carbs, they will fill you up until your next meal. So it's much easier to stick to the rest of this Candida diet food list and not give into naughty snack temptations. Say about yoghurt what you want but it's undeniable that it promotes bowel movements, which is a clear issue for most Candida sufferers. Too much info I know, but it had to be said!

**Cons for eating yoghurt and feta:**

One of the reasons why some people are completely against consuming dairy products is its specific protein structure, which makes it hard to digest for humans.
Yoghurt made from cow's milk can especially lead to bowel problems like loose stools and bloating in sensitive individuals. On the Candida diet, of course, you also have to worry about the remaining milk sugar in the dairy product that can still aggravate your yeast problem. Less so with goat's cheese than with milk, but still. Every little bit adds up.

**My experience with eating yoghurt and feta on the diet:**

I personally noticed that eating yoghurt or feta cheese at the beginning of Stage 3 did not agree with me very well at all (mainly more sinuses problems). It was months into Stage 3 that I noticed no problem when eating it.

These days, I stick to goat's/ sheep's yoghurt when I eat it and still limit myself to just a few spoonful's. By the way, there are huge differences in taste in goat's yoghurts (they are not all pungent and runny). I found one that is just like Greek yoghurt made by Woodland Dairy, and it is very mild and nice.

I avoid cow's milk/yoghurt altogether and I have just started making kefir from full fat goat's milk. Drinking half a glass up to twice a day helps me avoid a Candida relapse. You can also make it with water, rice milk, cow's milk or coconut milk.

Here's a tutorial on how you can make it at home www.candidadietplan.com/how-to-make-kefir/. Again, try a small amount first. You might not be able to tolerate a lot in the beginning (i.e., half a small glass or so). Mozzarella has a lot more milk sugar content than feta or kefir, and it is therefore more likely to cause you symptoms (e.g., a yeast infection flare up, bloating or cold-like symptoms).

**Conclusion: small amounts of yoghurt and feta, kefir or tofu are okay.**

If you eat yoghurt, feta or goat's cheese in Stage 2 of the diet, it is likely to cause you some symptoms, being it a sore throat, sneezing or nausea. It should agree better with you from Stage 3 on.
But listen to your body -- if you only have a mild yeast infection, then you might not have to be so cautious. This is more for people with food intolerances, who feel bloated or have a stuffy nose.

If you do decide to have some yoghurt, stick to no more than 4-6 tablespoons and don't eat it every day. Try it with desiccated coconut, sunflower seeds, cinnamon and puffed rice -- yum! Okay, it took me a while to grow to like it but your taste buds adapt, promise!

**All Veggies are Allowed**

- All of the Stage 2 veggies:
- Avocado
- Cucumbers, courgettes (zucchinis), celery
- Green and leafy vegetables (kale, spring greens/collard, chard, spinach, watercress, French beans, broccoli, handful of peas)
- Tomatoes, bell peppers, aubergine (eggplant)
- Salad (avoid the mixed pre-packed variety)
- Onions, leek, garlic
- Artichoke (keep Jerusalem artichokes to a minimum though for the time being as they can cause bloating and excess gas)
- Fennel, asparagus
- Chickpeas (they are actually a vegetable and not a bean, believe it or not)
- Fresh herbs (basil, coriander, mint, lemon balm)
- Sea vegetables/algae (nori, wakame, etc.)

**Plus root vegetables and starchy vegetables:**

- Carrots, beetroot, parsnips, pumpkin, butternut squash, corn

- Potatoes, turnips and any other vegetable you can think of
- Always combine these with green vegetables or salad and seeds to keep blood sugar levels constant
- Start with small amounts (e.g., 2 small potatoes) as a side dish and go from there to determine if this doesn't cause you more symptoms.
- If you experience symptoms, go back to Stage 2 foods and try again in 2-4 weeks.

- Choose cold cooked potatoes over baked potatoes due to their lower glycemic index levels (less sugar in your blood means less Candida risk).

**Plus fermented vegetables:**
Sauerkraut and kimchi (only 1-2 tablespoons at first, then gradually more)

**From Stage 3, the Candida diet food list also includes beans and lentils:**

- Butter beans, kidney beans, pinto beans, black-eyed peas
- Red lentils, green lentils, split peas
- Legumes and heart-warming soups make up a big part of our Candida diet food list because they are the ideal comfort food.
- Now you can also occasionally have chickpea flour dishes like onion bhajis (not too often though as fried foods are not good for you).

**Oils**

- Coconut oil
- Olive oil, organic sunflower oil or other oil of your choice
- Goat's butter/ghee
- Linseed oil (not for cooking)

**Stock and salad sauces, seasoning and spices:**

- Yeast-free stock cubes and homemade bone broth
- Coconut aminos

- Bragg's seasoning (non-fermented soya sauce)
- Organic tomato paste and tinned tomatoes (as long as it contains no citric acid)
- Low salt or sea salt, freshly ground black pepper, turmeric, cayenne pepper, ginger spice, garlic, thyme
- Organic spice mixes (e.g., mild curry)
- Creamed coconut
- Apple cider vinegar, olive oil and lemon juice
- Salad sauce made from lemon juice, stevia and yoghurt
- Cinnamon, vanilla
- Ground arrow root or organic beef gelatin for thickening

**Best baking ingredients**

- Ground almonds/almond flour, flaked almonds
- Coconut flour, desiccated coconut, flaxseeds
- Spelt flour or gluten free flour (can still cause you reactions)
- Rice milk/unsweetened almond milk/coconut milk/semi skimmed goat's milk
- Stevia

**Superfoods and protein powder for extra energy**

- Spirulina, chlorella, maca, barleygrass, hemp seeds are all very good.
- In terms of protein powder, go for hemp or pea protein (occasionally whey or soya).

**Allowed only once or twice per week**

- Cooked brown rice or quinoa (e.g., a big bowl full with coconut oil and cinnamon, chewed slowly)
- Probiotic yoghurt (a medium tub)
- Handful of sunflower seeds or pumpkin seeds

- Handful of nuts (preferably freshly cracked or soaked; almonds are best)

## Foodie tips for a gluten-free diet

Let's get this straight -- I think you should eat gluten-free, regardless of whether you have ever done so before the diet or not. It is simply easier on your digestive system, which speeds up your healing.

- Quinoa, buckwheat, millet or amaranth are back on the books for you now, yippee! It's best to rotate grains though. Stick to *50-75g (approx. 1/3 cup)*. Wash thoroughly, cook properly and eat only small amounts to avoid allergy symptoms. Brown rice agrees best with me. But it might be different for you.

I personally love spelt (so spelt flour is a definite for me for making bread -- a thousand times better for you than bread made from wheat). I know it's not suitable for those with celiac disease, but it is very low in gluten. So if you only had a Candida-induced grain intolerance, then chances are you can eat this happily in Stage 3.

- If you still feel bloated after eating spelt, ease off for a couple of weeks or longer and go back to the Candida diet food list for Stage 2 for the time being.
- Teff flour is a wonderful gluten-free dark rich flour (i.e., for tea cakes).
- You can use Bob's Red Mill All-Purpose Gluten-Free Flour for baking. Or you can mix your own, which is fun.
- And you can quickly whip up delicious almond flour buns or coconut flour muffins.

## Now we're talking bread – What are your options?

Your options are endless (at least compared to Stage 2). You can bake bread from any grain you like (except wheat is not recommended as it aggravates the gut and that's just what we set out to fight). Just don't use wheat. Even the healthy Ezekiel breads contain wheat, so watch out – unless of course wheat agrees with you.

## Sugar-free cakes and biscuits

Anything goes -- waffles, pancakes, muffins –
if you can bake it, you can make it! Just start s-l-o-w-l-y!
Start with one slice of yumminess and combine it with some anti-
Candida tea. Add cinnamon and flaked almonds or other nuts to
prevent your blood sugar from spiking. And be sure to put no
sugar, fruit or sweetener in it except stevia. Get aluminum-free
baking powder.

## Candida diet food list ideas for vegans:

In addition to the stage 2 type foods like green vegetables and co
you can also eat quinoa or any other grain you fancy (test small
amounts first to see if you're ready for it yet). In terms of baking,
you can easily adapt most bread/bun recipes that require egg to
include flaxseeds soaked in three times the amount of water (see
my Teff Bread recipe for instance
http://candidadietplan.com/vegan-teff-bread/ ). I would leave
tempeh as well as mushrooms and any other veggie meat
alternatives, such as Quorn, right until you are virtually symptom
free and you don't react to any of the other foods above anymore.

## Cereals/Breakfast

- Rice milk with puffed brown rice or other puffed grain are
  okay (flakes or bran of any kind are no good because they
  always contain some kind of sugar often disguised as malt
  something or other).
- Gluten-free porridge oats/oatmeal and quinoa are okay, as
  long as they agree with you. (Sadly, granola doesn't stick
  together without some form of sugar or dried fruit, so that's
  a no go.)
- Ground rice pudding or brown rice farina (Bob's Red Mill)
  with rice milk are lovely.
- Try to mix your breakies up with Stage 2 type breakies not to
  overdo the carbs. I had curried cabbage with sesame soda
  bread during the week and oatmeal porridge as a treat at the
  weekends. That worked very well for me.

## Pasta, pasta!

- Technically you can have whole wheat pasta.
  But I recommend you stick with gluten-free alternatives until you are fully restored to your former self.

- Rice pasta
- Quinoa pasta
- Corn pasta (the least healthy out of all of them)
- Soba noodles (i.e., made from buckwheat because it has the shortest cooking time)

Rice pasta agreed best with me. The other pasta types all caused symptoms in me. Try and see for yourself. It almost always agreed better with me when I had some cooked grains rather than pasta. But for a quick, easy to digest meal, these are unbeatable.

## Menu suggestions for Stage 3:

Not only vegetable omelettes, vegetable soup, chicken soup, steamed fish and grilled chicken breast from Stage 2. Now you can also enjoy rich lentil stews, beans, hot pots, pancakes and opulent breakfasts. Mild homemade vegetable and chicken curries, frittatas with potatoes and veggies, veggie stir-fry with feta or tempeh, baked potatoes with tuna, quinoa-beans salad… including a few desserts and sugar-free cakes…

## Try to eat mostly alkaline foods.
This will help you beat Candida faster. Alkaline foods are mostly salad and vegetables and almonds. In other words, balance your meat/ fish/ nuts intake with vegetables.

## List of hot drinks that are allowed on our yeast-free diet

- Green tea
- Chamomile peppermint tea (calms nerves and aids digestion)
- Ginger tea (double thumb size piece of ginger chopped and boiled in 1 liter+ of water)

## Hot detox drinks

- Hot water (cooking the water for 20 minutes or longer makes it alkaline, which is very good for you)
- Nettle mullein tea (good detox that combats cold symptoms, not sold in stores; you have to buy it loose and mix yourself)
- Hot lemon
- Dandelion root coffee (not the granules they contain sugar)
- Pau d'Arco tea

## List of cold drinks that you can drink

- Filtered water (lots of it!)
- Rice milk, coconut, soya and almond milk
- Apple cider vinegar (ACV) drink (2 teaspoons of cloudy ACV diluted in a glass of water -- drink upon awakening and before/with every meal, if you can stomach it; some people are sensitive and need to heal those areas first)
- Ice cold sparkling water with fresh lemon juice (refreshing summer drink)
- Green juice (glass of water with 1/2 teaspoon of chlorella powder and a hint of spirulina, with the option to add the juice from half a lemon)
- Lemonade with lime, lemon balm and stevia

*And before you know it, the Candida diet is over and you can enjoy your favorite sweet foods again. Hang in there!*

## What NOT to Eat/ Drink:

Basically, you are still avoiding pretty much the same foods as in Stage 2 - namely sugar, fruit and sweets of all kinds. This includes oats and wheat-based cereals, pasta and breads.

## Sweet foods

- Sugar, honey, agave, coconut sugar
- Fresh and dried fruit, jam, honey
- Chocolate and sweets
- Cakes, biscuits and other sweet bakery treats *(you can now eat cake without sugar/with stevia though!)*
- White flour *(also white pasta and egg noodles; you can now eat soba noodles and rice pasta though)*
- Big amounts of mushy starchy/sweet vegetables *(e.g., potato mash, beetroot, sweet potatoes, parsnips)*
- Muesli with dried fruit -- hard to digest and full of sugar
- Packaged cereal *(e.g., wheat flakes, bran, rice crispies)* except for unsweetened puffed cereals

## Fermented or containing additives

- Cheese *(except feta and small amounts of mozzarella)*
- Mushrooms
- Stock cubes with yeast
- Bread with yeast, banana or sugar in any form. Sourdough bread isn't good either unfortunately *(even natural yeast causes symptoms)*
- Battered food including scotch eggs, fish or sausages
- Anything containing fermented food like soya sauce, miso soup, vinegar *(with the exception of apple cider vinegar)*
- Canned foods with citric acid (e.g., tomatoes or coconut milk if half of the content is guar gum or other additives; go for organic just water added)

## Foods that are difficult to digest

- Hot spicy sauces, deep fried food and red meats

## Foods that could cause an allergic response

- Oats/wheat
- Nuts (unless freshly cracked)
- Sweetener

## Drinks that are not permitted

- Coffee (stimulants make the body release sugar reserves into the blood stream as readily available energy; the dirty little scoundrels can even feed on that, if you can believe that)
- Alcohol
- Milk (contains milk sugars and is mucous producing)
- Fruit juices (even freshly squeezed!) and smoothies
- Lemonade, energy drinks
- Kombucha (fermented tea that, due to its acidic and mildly alcoholic nature, is not ideal for Candida sufferers until virtually no symptoms are present)

## You can have some filling snacks to tame your cravings though:

What use would a Candida diet food list be without at least a few snacks when you get ravenous?!

## Here are a few quick, filling treats for you to try:
(It's best to mix and match; try to keep carbs still at a minimum.)

- Avocado
- Green Smoothie
- Hummus and veggie sticks (preferably make your own hummus; if not, then buy organic)
- Freshly cracked nuts and seeds
- Rice milk with desiccated coconut flakes, sunflower seeds and cinnamon
- Cooked brown rice or quinoa with coconut oil
- Chicken soup
- Lightly spiced and fried green veg with toasted seeds and sesame oil
- 2 brown rice cakes with linseed oil and nori
- Probiotic yoghurt with vanilla, cinnamon, sunflower seeds, linseed oil and puffed rice
- Sesame soda bread with almond butter or coconut oil
- Gluten-free porridge oats with rice milk, cinnamon and shelled hemp seeds (Eat this once a week, if it agrees with you;

from my experience, you'll heal quicker the less grains you eat. I say that with a tear in my eyes since I LOVE porridge, granola, breads...).

**Five not-so-healthy snacks that are just about allowed on our Candida diet food List once in a while:**

- Corn cakes, popcorn (1-2 corn cakes/a handful of popcorn)
- Puffed rice
- Nachos, tacos (in moderation -- well as far as possible; aim for no more than 2 helpings )
- Instant quinoa or millet flakes with rice milk, almond milk or coconut milk
- Carob chocolate (no more than 1-2 pieces)

**Why are there no chocolate snacks on this Candida diet food list? Not even from dark cocoa?**

It might not have any sugar in it but since cocoa stimulates your adrenals, it triggers your body to release sugar from your cells into the blood stream where it can encourage Candida to grow.

It also plays havoc with your biological clock, overriding your feeling of tiredness, zapping up nutrients and bringing the digestive processes to a standstill, and promoting constipation, which in turn can trigger more Candida. Not to mention that you'd be craving more sweets, coffee and tea very quickly to maintain the elated feeling the chocolate snack gives you.

That's why I don't include any homemade cocoa snacks in this Candida diet food list, although they are of course delicious, healthy and ideal to curb your appetite and elevate your mood. Now you know, and there's no reason you couldn't enjoy a piece of good quality dark chocolate every once in a while instead of store-bought sweets. Just not ALL the time!

## Tips against Cravings:

Your body is particularly craving sweet things when your magnesium levels are low. So a good start is to eat some ***brown rice, nuts, almonds, green vegetables or take a magnesium supplement (for women especially before their period).***

## Quick Snack Tip:

For the time being you just have to be prepared for your cravings and eat foods that fill you up and are as healthy as possible (**e.g.,** ***spicy chickpeas*** - lightly heated up with olive oil, salt, pepper and garlic granules are a good quick filler for instance if you think you can't handle your cravings any longer).

## Quick and comforting Snacks:

- Rice milk with sunflower seeds and shredded coconut
- Toasted bread with almond butter or coconut oil
- Fresh or toasted pancakes (combine with green juice)
- Soba noodles with sesame oil and a pinch of salt
- Instant or pre-cooked quinoa/millet flakes with almond, rice or coconut milk
- A piece of carob chocolate as an emergency

## Healthier Snacks:

- Yogurt with puffed rice and cinnamon
- Rice cakes with flax oil and nori or sauerkraut

# Best snacks:

- Avocado
- Bone broth or chicken soup
- Cucumber slices
- Green juice or smoothie
- Leftovers from sweet potato and greens with salt, pepper and flax oil

- Brown rice with coconut oil or with rice milk and cinnamon
- Boiled egg and a bit of steamed veg
- My Simple Stir-Fry:

Steam some chopped spring greens, and cabbage or broccoli for a few minutes. Then lightly fry them in a bit of spice (e.g., salt, pepper, turmeric, ginger, cayenne) with some leek. Coconut oil or sesame oil work well. Sprinkle with sesame seeds and toss around to mix with spice and oil. Continue frying for a moment. Great snack, also nice with a bit of freshly grated carrot thrown in at the end of cooking.

Did you know that I upload new Candida diet friendly recipes to my blog nearly every week? You might just find the meal you're craving at the moment.

Head over to http://candidadietplan.com/best-candida-diet-recipes/ and check out my mean Healing Breakfast and Thai Green Curry

## Smoothies:

### Creamy Green Calmer Smoothie

- 5 lettuce leaves
- ½ one cucumber
- 1 handful of spinach
- Chlorella
- Spirulina
- 1 handful of cashew nuts
- ½ can chilled creamy coconut milk
- Rice milk
- optional: handful of fresh coriander, basil or mint leaves

Simply blend all the ingredients until you have a thick and creamy smoothie. The name says it all -- this smoothie really calms you down. And if it brings a moment of calm to your day, that can only be good, right? Now, I could tell you that's because of the *soporific* qualities of the lettuce.

But let's just say that once you experience the *silky sweet smoothness* of this coconutty creation, you'll forget all finer details anyway. The cashew nuts make this smoothie extra sweet and creamy.

**Simple Green Almond Smoothie**

- glass of unsweetened almond milk
- 1 whole cucumber, peeled and cubed
- 1 flax egg (1 tablespoon flaxseeds soaked in 3 tablespoons water for 10 minutes)
- 2 tablespoons ground almonds
- ½ teaspoon chlorella
- Optional: 1 tablespoon protein powder for an extra protein kick (I used whey)

Prepare the flax egg at least 15 minutes before you make your smoothie (soak 1 tablespoon of freshly ground flax seeds in 3-4 tablespoons of water). Add the liquids to your blender. Then the chopped cucumber, the powder and spices. Blend. Enjoy!

You can also enjoy the Simple Coconut Smoothie from Stage 2 or other smoothies with similar ingredients.

# Why you need Probiotics:

**You need Probiotics to strengthen your Gut and Immune System**

Probiotics, such as L.acidophilus, are responsible for creating a healthy balance of *'friendly bacteria'* in your gut.

They are beneficial live microorganisms that basically build a protective layer in your body by lining your intestines. That's how they prevent harmful substances from getting into your bloodstream. Since *more than 70 percent of the body's immune system is based in the gut*, these friendly little helpers are fairly important.

When your count of probiotics is low, this results in digestive upsets as you are lacking essential enzymes to break down food. You might also get ill, as the naturally occurring harmful bacteria in your body are not kept in check. Hence you're now battling with Candida. But all is not lost! You can boost your health by eating foods that are naturally high in probiotics like sauerkraut or kefir.

It is well worth learning to make your own fermented probiotic foods. Then you can slowly phase out the expensive probiotic supplements you have been taking.

There's a free tutorial on how to do this on my blog http://candidadietplan.com/how-to-make-sauerkraut/

## Probiotics and Candida – when should you start taking them?

The idea is to *start with a low dose of probiotics (around 5 billion CFU) about 2-3 weeks into the diet (at the beginning of Stage 3)*, when your body is already accustomed to taking antifungal remedies.

You can start the probiotics at the same time as the antifungals *(at a different time of day though)*. It doesn't hurt to take them earlier *(as in during the cleanse)*. It's just a bit of a waste though, because you are flushing out your intestines with the cleanse.

It's generally *recommended to start the probiotics a couple of weeks after you've started on the antifungals* as the probiotics will also cause a die-off reaction, and you might end up feeling ill. It's best to start slowly, so your body can get used to it.

Then you work your way up to a higher dose of *20-50 billion CFU*. And if your immune system has been taken a proper knock, you might even have to take probiotics as strong as *100 billion CFU*. But don't let that concern you when you first start the Candida diet. Initially, you don't need to take a probiotic supplement at all.

If you were to take high strength probiotics, this would most likely over-burden your liver and make you sick.

*Even natural probiotics, such as kefir or yoghurt, are generally not well tolerated initially. They can cause you sniffles, a sore throat or give you a slight feeling of nausea.*

And even when you decide to re-introduce yoghurt (unpasteurized and unsweetened) 2-3 weeks into the Candida diet, go easy on it.

Start with no more than 2 tablespoons and work your way up to more if you don't experience any side effects. The last thing you need now is some allergy symptoms on top of everything else!

The easiest yoghurt to digest is sheep's yoghurt *(and it doesn't even smell as if a goat had breathed in your face like goat's yoghurts generally do, ha!).*

*Take them at least 3 hours apart from your antifungals.*

For instance, you could take them *first thing in the morning 20 minutes before breakfast and again before your dinner with a big glass of cold water (hot liquid or acidic foods can kill some of the goodness).*

## How long do you need to take them?

Many people feel so much better from taking probiotics that they are reluctant to stop taking them for fear of getting ill again. Especially if you are leading a hectic lifestyle, it can be a good idea to take probiotics preventatively to support your immune system. That said, I am a firm believer in real food and feel that, given a chance, the body becomes strong enough to keep Candida in check on its own.

I think once you have treated your digestive issues, removed any allergens and created some balance in your life whilst enjoying a varied diet with fermented vegetables, you won't need to take supplements anymore.

**Here's a list of reputable probiotics brands:**

- MegaFlora from MegaFoods (US)
- Flora from Innate Response (US)
- Ultimate Flora Probiotics from Renew Life (US)
- Garden Of Life's Primal Defense Ultra (US/ UK)
- Custom Probiotics CP-1 from Immunecare.co.uk (UK)
- Optibac Probiotics extra Strength (UK)
- ProbioMax DF from Xymogen (US)
- HMF Neuro Probiotics by Genestra (Rockwell Nutrition) (US)

**What Probiotics I've Taken:**

- Probio Intensive *(9 billion CFUs per capsule, 3 strains)*

- Optibac Probiotics for daily well-being *(2.5 billion per capsule, 6 different strains which included 88 mg prebiotics).*
- Optibacs Extra Strength Probiotic *(20 billion CFUs; just without the prebiotics)*
- Garden Of Life's Primal Defense Ultra *(15 billion CFUs, 13 strains)* – High Quality Broad Spectrum Soil Based Probiotics.
- Custom Probiotics CP-1 from Immunecare.co.uk *(78 billion CFUs, 5 strains)* – This is a great probiotic supplement for clearing skin and allergy issues.

**Start with a low dose of probiotics. Then gradually take stronger ones until you are virtually symptom free.**

Then start to eat additional probiotic and prebiotic foods *(think probiotic yoghurt and kefir; cabbage, leek, onions, Jerusalem artichokes)*.

And gradually take fewer supplements until you have reached a level that you are personally comfortable with.

### Symptoms

You will encounter the same or similar symptoms as in Stage 2 of the diet. So use the symptoms checklist from chapter 2 and the home remedies I've given you in chapter 3 for reference.

## Recap of Stage 3: Boost your immune system with Probiotics

You're *rebuilding your gut*'s *health with probiotics*, which in turn boosts your immune system. Win-Win! You're also continuing to *heal any food intolerances, grain sensitivities* or any other symptoms and learn what healthy snacks you can have to tame your cravings.

# CHAPTER FIVE
## TRANSITION BACK TO NORMAL EATING

### Why you can't get back to your old eating habits

You can't just go back to your old eating habits because *your immune system is not yet strong enough* and you would get a Candida relapse if you ate like you did before. By the end of Stage 4 though, your immune system should be strong enough to control the Candida itself without any help.

### What you need to do:

You'll still need to continue following a sugar-free diet for a whole year. Now is the time to try all those foods that used to cause you symptoms when you started the diet (e.g., fruit, fermented foods, etc.) Also, you still have to take a strong probiotic to help your immune system deal with this new way of eating.

**What You Can Eat (but should still only enjoy occasionally for the time being)**

- Bread made with yeast, fruit, cow's milk and yoghurt
- Cakes sweetened half with stevia and the other half with Xylitol (a diabetic friendly sweetener that contains a small amount fruit sugar which makes it forbidden in the beginning of the diet)
- Even foods that naturally rebalance your gut like Sauerkraut and Jerusalem artichokes (eat often if it agrees with you – just be aware that it can cause bloating or gas initially)
- Fermented foods like vinegar, cheese, soy sauce, pickles or sauces
- Tempeh as well as mushrooms, nutritional yeast and any other veggie meat alternatives, such as Quorn

Obviously, the idea is not to try any of those last foods unless you actually want to eat them -- and not unless you actually feel good. Bear in mind that these foods might still cause you symptoms. *So it's worth taking it really slowly and if in doubt, just stick to the foods you know agree with you* -- even if it means eating mostly Stage 2 and 3 foods. Why take risks if you don't have to? After all, you have probably become used to your healthy sugar-free diet now, haven't you?!

So as soon as you are symptom free and you don't need any antifungal supplements anymore, you can start experimenting with the foods above. But don't go all overboard with this. Add *no more than one new food per week* to see if you react to it. If you eat it all at once, then it's impossible to tell what might have caused your reaction. In this transition stage, *you can now start eating fruit again.* Yay!

But be careful. Start with only a few slices of fruit, rather than the whole fruit. For instance, you can start by adding some pieces of frozen fruit to smoothies; say half a small apple or a handful of blueberries.

**Here's a great smoothie with a little fruit to get you started:**

**Creamy Calmer Smoothie with fruit**

- 4 small green organic lettuce leaves
- 3 heaped tablespoons coconut milk
- almond milk (just a little)
- 1 heaped teaspoon chia seeds
- 2 teaspoons cashew nuts
- celery
- ½ mini apple
- ½ teaspoon chlorella
- optional: 2 tablespoons unpasteurized yoghurt/soya yoghurt (I used sheep's yoghurt which is milder than goats' yoghurt, similar to Greek yoghurt)
- optional: ½ organic lemon

Soak the chia seeds in three times as much water for 15-20 minutes. Chop the apple and celery, and blend with all the other ingredients until you are left with a creamy smoothie consistency.

**Cathy's Key Lime Pie Smoothie -- Favorite Reader's Recipe!**

- ¼ cup coconut milk
- ¼ cup plain non pasteurized yoghurt
- 3 sticks celery
- 1 whole cucumber
- 1 whole lime
- 1 granny smith apple (take out the seeds)
- handful of spinach
- pinch of kale
- optional: ¼ cup buckwheat or flax

Juice all. Blend ¼ cup coconut milk and ¼ cup plain unpasteurized yoghurt into juice. Then add the buckwheat or flax.

**And you can also enjoy:**

- *The odd bit of carob or dark chocolate.*
- You can even have *desserts* again.

- You can make snack bars from *cereal, lightly sweetened by agave nectar or coconut sugar.*
- At family gatherings or birthday bashes, you can enjoy a *glass of wine or a big slice of cream gateaux cake* (okay, make that 2 slices…)
- And you go to a beach barbecue and slap *ketchup* on your burger or even take a big bite out of a white burger bun.

All these things are okay, as long as you do only one food experiment per week and you go back to a clean diet for the rest of the week. Every week.

**P.S.: More food ideas coming your way.** I constantly share tons of tasty recipes on the *Candida Diet Plan Facebook page:*

*https://www.facebook.com/CandidaDietPlan?ref=hl*
*on Twitter @candidadiettips*
and on *Pinterest http://pinterest.com/sandraboehner/.*
*Come and connect with me!*

**What you can't eat:**

- You can't eat anything with *cane sugar, highly processed foods or foods with lots of additives.*
- You shouldn't be eating *wheat, especially white bread and white pasta and preferably not white rice either.*
- Try to avoid *coffee, chocolate, cereal bars and take away food.*
- It's also best not to have *milk, cream, cheese or butter* on a regular basis.
- For the next 6-12 months, I would also still *avoid sweets, coffee and overly sweet fruit like dates, mango and bananas on a regular basis.* Or if you use it, eat only a few pieces rather than a whole fruit.

This will give your immune system a proper chance to re-establish a healthy balance.

## Recap of stage 4: Time to Eat Nice Foods Again!

Continue to *strengthen your immune system* by following a clean diet most of the time. You *reintroduce fermented foods, dairy and grains* to see if they agree with you now. Then you go back to your diet to solidify your health foundation. And whenever you do continue to react to certain foods, you go back to taking antifungals and natural remedies. That way, you ensure to *prevent a relapse and slowly get used to sweeter foods again.*

# Final Words

Congratulations!

You have made it through to the end. Ready to get started with the actual Candida diet?

**I'd love you to go to my website http://candidadietplan.com**

When you sign up for my newsletter you'll get access to four handy Candida diet food lists that you can print for easy reference - one for every stage of the diet. And you'll also **get my latest recipes and diet info sent to you by email.**

Thank you for reading my book!

I wish you the best of health & happiness,
Sandra Boehner

# SANDRA BOEHNER

When first diagnosed with a Candida and gluten intolerance, Sandra Boehner started creating sugar and gluten-free foods that helped her manage her health problems.

Through diet and natural treatments, she overcame Candida, eczema, thyroidism, depression, sinus infections and recurring yeast infections, amongst other health conditions.

At one point, Sandra suffered from eczema and allergies so severe that 90 percent of her body was covered with severe inflammation that could have been mistaken for third degree burns.

The Candida diet plan helped her heal all the infections and sensitivities in her body. During this period, she started www.candidadietplan.com, a blog devoted to helping people reverse their food allergies and Candida-inflicted health conditions.

She now lives in Cornwall (UK) with her partner, Johnny.

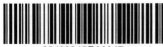

Printed in Poland
by Amazon Fulfillment
Poland Sp. z o.o., Wrocław